AN INNOVATIVE APPROACH TO LASTING

WEIGHT LOSS

Strategies for Sustainable Weight Transformation

DR JOYCE A. MOORE

This book does not offer psychiatric or medical advice; it is just intended for informational and educational purposes. If you have specific concerns about your medical or mental health, please speak with a trained expert.

amazon.com/author/joyceamoore

Copyright © 2023 by Dr Joyce A. Moore

Writing ***An Innovative Approach to Lasting Weight Loss*** has been a journey filled with learning, growth, and the unwavering support of so many incredible people.

First and foremost, I want to thank my readers—whether you're just starting your weight loss journey, searching for a new approach, or supporting someone you love. Your commitment to change and your willingness to explore new possibilities inspire me. This book is for you, and I hope it empowers you to embrace sustainable transformation with confidence.

To my family and friends, thank you for your endless encouragement, patience, and belief in me. Your support has been my anchor through the late nights, countless rewrites, and moments of doubt. You've reminded me that perseverance is the key to success—whether in writing or in health.

A special thanks to the experts, mentors, and researchers whose work has shaped the insights in this book. Your dedication to science, wellness, and human potential continues to make a lasting impact, and I am grateful to stand on the shoulders of giants.

To everyone who has ever shared their personal struggles, breakthroughs, and triumphs with me—your stories are a testament to resilience and the power of small, consistent changes. They have shaped this book in more ways than I can express.

Finally, to those who pick up this book and take even one small step toward a healthier, happier life—thank you. Your journey is yours alone, but you are never truly alone. I am honored to be a part of it.

With gratitude,

DR JOYCE A. MOORE

CONTENT

This is an innovative path towards achieving lasting weight loss. This book is not just another diet plan or fleeting trend; it's a holistic approach designed to transform your relationship with food, exercise, and self-care. Embracing a blend of scientific insights and practical strategies, this guide is tailored to fit into your unique lifestyle, offering sustainable methods to shed pounds and maintain a healthier and stronger body.

We investigate the psychology underlying our eating patterns, identifying triggers and laying the groundwork for mindful consuming by going beyond simple calorie tracking or rigid routines. Exercise becomes pleasurable and adaptive, rather than a job, as we find individualized fitness regimens based on individual interests and schedules. Furthermore, this approach emphasizes mental well-being, acknowledging the critical relationship between a healthy mind and a healthy body.

Learn to navigate challenges, setbacks, and plateaus with resilience, fostering a long-term commitment to a balanced, nourishing lifestyle. Get ready to embark on a transformative journey that goes beyond quick fixes, empowering you to achieve sustainable, lasting weight loss. The goal of this life-changing adventure is to redefine wellbeing rather than just lose weight. It ultimately boils down to accepting gradual, incremental adjustments that add up to big improvements.

Learn to plan your meals so that you may create enticing, healthful meals that will satisfy your palate and nourish your body. In order to create a fitness regimen that is sustainable and fits into your lifestyle, discover the joy of movement through a variety of training options that corresponds with your hobbies. It's time to embrace a healthier, happier you for long-lasting transformation, equipped with useful advice and a deeper comprehension of your body's demands.

There are several reasons why one feels constantly hungry, and they go beyond just a basic desire for food. Hormonal imbalance is one major factor, particularly ghrelin, which is sometimes referred to as the "hunger hormone." Changes in ghrelin levels can set off hunger signals, which force the body to search for food regardless of real energy needs.

In addition, insufficient sleep throws off the equilibrium of hormones that control appetite, increasing ghrelin and decreasing leptin, the hormone that indicates fullness. Stress, a common companion in modern life, causes the release of cortisol, which increases hunger and may cause emotional eating habits.

Another important factor is the makeup of the diet. Processed, high-sugar foods can rise and plummet blood sugar levels quickly, making you feel hungry shortly after eating. In a similar vein, inadequate consumption of fiber and protein does not maintain fullness, leading to repeated episodes of hunger.

Dehydration can masquerade as hunger, confusing signals within the body. Often, a glass of water can alleviate feelings of hunger, highlighting the importance of staying adequately hydrated.

Understanding these triggers empowers individuals to address hunger cues effectively. A balanced diet, sufficient sleep, stress management, and hydration constitute crucial elements in managing perpetual hunger. By recognizing these factors, individuals can adopt strategies that nourish the body effectively, curbing the sensation of constant hunger and promoting a more balanced relationship with food.

HOW TO EAT TO BEAT FAT

Embarking on a journey to shed excess fat isn't about deprivation—it's about making informed, enjoyable food choices that fuel your body and support lasting change. Let us explore how you can eat to beat fat effectively

Embrace Whole, Unprocessed Foods

Opt for foods in their natural state, such as fresh fruits, vegetables, lean proteins, whole grains, and healthy fats. These nutrient-dense options provide essential vitamins and minerals without the added sugars and unhealthy fats found in processed foods. Incorporating a variety of these foods can help you feel satisfied and energized while supporting weight loss.

Prioritize Protein Intake

Including adequate protein in your meals can boost metabolism, reduce appetite, and help preserve muscle mass during weight loss. Aim to incorporate sources like lean meats, fish, legumes, dairy products, and plant-based proteins into your diet. For example, Greek yogurt is a high-protein option that can keep you feeling full and satisfied.

Choose High-Fiber Foods

Foods rich in fiber, such as whole grains, legumes, fruits, and vegetables, aid digestion and promote a feeling of fullness, helping to control hunger and reduce overall calorie intake. For instance, incorporating quinoa into your meals adds both fiber and protein, supporting your weight loss efforts.

Incorporate Healthy Fats

Not all fats are created equal. Healthy fats, like those found in avocados, nuts, seeds, and olive oil, can promote satiety and support overall health. Including these in moderation can help you feel full longer and reduce the likelihood of overeating.

Be Mindful of Carbohydrate Quality and Timing

Focus on consuming complex carbohydrates with a low glycemic index, such as whole grains and legumes, which provide sustained energy and help regulate blood sugar levels. Timing your carbohydrate intake around physical activity can also optimize energy utilization and fat burning.

Stay Hydrated

Drinking sufficient water is crucial for overall health and can aid in weight loss by promoting satiety and supporting metabolic processes. Sometimes, our bodies can misinterpret thirst as hunger, leading to unnecessary calorie consumption.

Practice Mindful Eating

Pay attention to your body's hunger and fullness cues, eat slowly, and savor your meals. This practice can prevent overeating and help you develop a healthier relationship with food.

Remember, the goal is to create a balanced and enjoyable eating pattern that you can maintain in the long term. By making these thoughtful food choices, you're not just losing fat—you're nourishing your body and setting the foundation for a healthier future.

An endless desire for food is frequently caused by a complex interaction of environmental, psychological, and physiological variables. The complex web of hormones and neurotransmitters that controls appetite and satiety is at the heart of it. The "hunger hormone," ghrelin, peaks before meals and decreases thereafter. It varies throughout the day. Persistent desires, however, might be brought on by disturbances in its rhythm, which may result from erratic eating patterns or insufficient sleep. Triggers that are psychological and emotional also have a big impact. An urge for food may be sparked by boredom, stress, anxiety, or even habit. Mindless eating as a coping strategy is very frequently the result. Emotional cues blend in with learned habits, forming connections between feelings or circumstances and the need to eat even in the absence of physical hunger.

Dietary choices can exacerbate cravings. Highly processed, sugary, or high-fat foods can hijack the brain's reward system, fostering addictive tendencies that perpetuate cravings. Moreover, inadequate nutrient intake, especially essential nutrients like protein or fiber, can leave the body seeking more sustenance, leading to persistent hunger.

Environmental cues play a pivotal role as well. Surrounded by food advertisements, easy access to snacks, and social influences, the brain receives constant signals triggering cravings, even when not genuinely hungry.

Understanding these multifaceted triggers is key to managing persistent food cravings. Cultivating mindfulness around eating habits, addressing emotional triggers, nourishing the body with balanced meals, and creating a supportive environment that minimizes exposure to tempting foods are crucial steps toward regaining control over cravings. By adopting strategies that address these various aspects, individuals can develop a healthier relationship with food, breaking the cycle of constant cravings and promoting a more balanced approach to eating.

Regaining control over eating habits is possible for people who learn to manage these triggers. Recognizing the multifaceted nature of cravings for junk food allows for a more comprehensive approach toward healthier choices. Satiety and general well-being are enhanced by incorporating a well-balanced diet full of nutrient-dense foods, emphasizing enough sleep, practicing stress management techniques, and ensuring you drink enough water. By adopting these holistic strategies, individuals can effectively navigate the complexities of perpetual cravings, fostering a harmonious connection with food that supports physical health and emotional and mental balance.

The biological, psychological, and environmental elements that combine to produce a strong desire for these less nourishing but very appetizing options are frequently the cause of junk food cravings. The reward system in the brain has a major biological influence. Junk food triggers dopamine pathways, which results in feelings of reward and pleasure. Junk food is usually heavy in sugar, fat, and salt. As the brain looks for the recognizable dopamine spike that comes from eating these foods, this might eventually cause cravings. Furthermore, cultural and environmental factors are quite important. Cravings are encouraged by social norms surrounding the consumption of junk food, simple accessibility, and ubiquitous advertising. In addition to social cues, the sight or scent of certain foods alone might pique someone's interest and lead to consumption.

Additionally, the appeal of junk food is influenced by conditioning and habit. Frequent consumption creates brain connections that link specific stimuli—such as the sight or smell of fried food—to the enjoyment of eating. It is difficult to reject temptations when appetites are reinforced by these well-established behaviors.

There are several tactics involved in addressing these desires. Recalibrating the brain's reward system and lowering cravings can be accomplished by practicing mindfulness around triggers, finding alternate ways to manage stress, progressively minimizing exposure to unhealthy foods, and gradually introducing healthier alternatives for junk food. The goal is to retrain the environment and the mind to choose healthy options over quick satisfaction.

Real hunger is a physiological need for sustenance, as opposed to emotional or habitual needs. Comprehending and recognizing the actual hunger sign is essential for mindful eating and general health. Real hunger is characterized by a gradual onset that signals the body's desire for food rather than happening all at once. A growling stomach, a hollow or empty feeling, and perhaps a minor decrease in energy are examples of physical symptoms. Another important point to remember is that true hunger isn't food-specific; rather, it's a universal need for sustenance. It takes attentiveness to learn the difference between true hunger and other urges. It's important to take a moment to stop and evaluate your body's signals before grabbing food. It entails becoming aware of and in tune with the body's sensations without passing judgment and determining if the need to eat is a result of a true physiological requirement or other factors like boredom or stress. Recognizing trends and distinguishing real hunger cues can be aided by keeping a food diary or writing hunger levels and related feelings.

Examining the body's signals takes some thought and awareness. The secret is to be aware of how hunger differs for each individual. Some people may feel empty or have a growling stomach, while others may notice a decrease in energy. Understanding these cues makes it easier to distinguish between true hunger and other types of stimuli, such as emotional or habitual desires.

In the end, feeding on nutritious, well-balanced meals in response to these signs is the best way to acknowledge true hunger. A healthy connection with food may be fostered by those who recognize and honor their body's cues, which will support not just physical satiety but also emotional and mental well-being. Furthermore, taking into account the time of the previous meal is necessary to com prehend the body's hunger cues. A normal cycle of digestion and energy use is indicated by the emergence of true hunger many hours after eating. This hunger builds gradually and doesn't go away with activities or diversions;

it will continue to exist until enough food is given.

By developing a conscious interpretation of these signals, people may react to hunger cues in a way that gives their bodies the nourishment they require. Adopting this eating strategy promotes a healthy connection with food and supports both mental and physical health.

Creating a customized meal plan is a critical first step in keeping up a healthy, balanced diet that accommodates personal tastes and advances general health objectives. Evaluate your nutritional requirements and objectives first. Take into account variables such as the number of calories needed each day, the proportions of macronutrients (carbs, fats, and proteins), and any dietary limitations or preferences. Maintain portion control to ensure that you have three main meals a day and, if necessary, add in nutritious snacks.

Begin by organizing meals around whole, high-nutrient foods. Make a point of including complete grains, lean meats, vibrant fruits and veggies, and healthy fats. Changing up the cooking techniques and taste profiles you use may provide variety and enjoyment to your meals.

Plan your meals according to normal meal times to ensure that you have steady energy levels all day. Try to eat three major meals a day, and if necessary, add in some nutritious snacks. Just remember to watch your portion sizes to align with your goals.

It's important to plan ahead. Set aside a particular day of the week to prepare meals. Preparing ingredients or full meals ahead of time will help you stay on track when things become busy. Make a shopping list that takes into account the meals you have planned so you know you have everything you need.

Adaptability is essential. Make space for modifications and alterations due to shifting plans or unanticipated events. Accept flexibility without sacrificing the dishes' overall nutritional balance.

Monitor your development and see how your body reacts to various food combinations. Consult a nutritionist or dietitian for advice on creating a food plan that suits your individual requirements and health goals.

Beyond simply choosing foods, creating a great meal plan requires careful thought into several important factors. It involves establishing a framework that is durable and fits your preferences, way of life, and health goals. It's critical to comprehend portion sizes and practice mindful eating. A well-rounded meal is ensured by arranging the right amounts of proteins, carbs, and fats on your plate. Including foods from a range of food, categories give your meals more variety and enjoyment in addition to providing necessary nutrients.

Keeping your meal plan flexible allows you to be spontaneous without sacrificing structure. Periodically straying is okay as long as it doesn't interfere with your overall dietary objectives. Accept moderation and balance above strict regulations.

Investigation and experimenting are crucial to keep your meal plan interesting and avoid boredom, explore possibilities with different recipes, cuisines, and ingredients. It makes it possible to find healthier substitutions or alternatives that fit your dietary needs and preferences.

Smart grocery shopping is another aspect of meal planning. Make fresh, natural meals your top priority while shopping, and steer clear of excessively processed foods. Having a well-stocked pantry with various items means you'll always have alternatives for dinner preparation.

Finally, sustainability is essential. A long-term food plan should be manageable and pleasurable to stick to. Eating the foods you enjoy in moderation reduces feelings of deprivation and increases the likelihood that you will follow through on your plan.

Setting up a meal plan that is flexible and consistent can help you develop a healthy eating pattern that benefits your general health. Review and adjust your food plan regularly as necessary to ensure it meets your nutritional needs and lifestyle changes.

HOW TO OVERCOME DIFFICULTIES WITH WEIGHT LOSS CHALLENGES

Overcoming obstacles to weight loss frequently calls for a multidimensional strategy that takes into account aspects more than just food and exercise.

First and foremost, it's critical to comprehend and control expectations. It's quite common for weight loss efforts to have plateaus or slower progress at times. Motivation may be sustained with persistence, patience, and an emphasis on total health gains rather than simply the numbers on the scale.

It might be helpful to recognize and treat underlying causes that affect weight. This includes elements that might impede development, such as stress, poor sleep, hormone imbalances, or underlying medical issues. Consulting with healthcare experts, such as dietitians, physicians, or therapists, can yield insightful advice and customized tactics.

The key to sustainability is redesigning your lifestyle, rather than relying on temporary solutions. This includes incorporating reasonable and modest dietary adjustments. Long-term success is enhanced by implementing realistic, progressive improvements in stress management, exercise regimens, and food habits. Accept a healthy, whole-food-based diet that fits your lifestyle and is well-balanced.

Putting in place a support network may have a big impact. As you pursue your objectives, surround yourself with people who support and encourage you—whether that means friends, family, or joining wellness and health-focused communities. Support groups or accountability partners can provide encouragement and direction when things are tough.

Stress reduction methods and mindful eating are useful strategies. Overeating causes may be managed by exercising portion control, understanding the difference between actual hunger and emotional desires, and utilizing stress-relieving techniques like yoga or meditation.

Lastly, it's critical to reframe failures as teaching moments. Honor all advancement, no matter how small, and learn from challenges along the way. Acknowledge all of your accomplishments, and take lessons from your mistakes. A positive outlook and self-compassion are crucial for long-term success during the weight loss process. Remember that maintaining a better, happier lifestyle is just as important as losing weight in a sustainable way.

EATING AGAINST YOUR OWN DESIRE

Eating against one's desires frequently results from engaging in a way that is inconsistent with what one needs or wants. There are several reasons for this discordance, such as entrenched behaviors, societal influences, or emotional triggers.

Emotional eating is a widespread phenomenon in which people use food as a coping method for boredom, stress, depression, or even joy. Eating is not a response to bodily hunger but rather an attempt to satiate an emotional need. To deal with these emotional triggers, one must learn to be aware of how they feel and create appropriate ways to cope that prevent overindulging in food. Social and environmental factors are also quite important. Eating habits might be influenced by cultural norms, peer pressure, or society standards. Social events and festivities, For instance, social gatherings or celebrations often revolve around food, leading individuals to eat not out of personal desire but due to societal expectations or to blend in with the group.

Eating patterns are also shaped by habits and taught actions. Mindless eating can result from ingrained habits or links between particular activities and eating, such as grabbing fast food on the run or munching while watching TV. These behaviors might occur even when one is not truly hungry.

Taking on these patterns calls for a diversified strategy. It entails recognizing emotional triggers, practicing alternate coping strategies, and becoming more attentive of one's eating behaviors. It's critical to foster an atmosphere that supports making better decisions and to practice self-compassion while facing difficulties.

In addition, cultivating a healthy relationship with food entails paying attention to internal signals rather than outside stimuli, eating mindfully, and respecting real hunger signals. People may take back control of their eating patterns and create a healthy lifestyle by coordinating their behaviors with their actual requirements and wants. Moreover, a lack of understanding about personal nutritional needs or relying on fad diets can contribute to eating against one's desires. This disconnect arises from not being in tune with the body's cues and nutritional requirements, leading to choices that don't align with genuine physical needs.

Addressing these issues involves cultivating a more profound connection with oneself and food. It entails fostering body acceptance, rejecting harmful dieting mentalities, and seeking nutritional education to make informed choices. Developing a mindful approach to eating, wherein individuals tune into their body's signals, fosters a more intuitive and authentic relationship with food.

Embracing a holistic view of health that encompasses mental, emotional, and physical well-being can facilitate aligning actions with genuine desires. By dismantling societal pressures, understanding individual nutritional needs, and nurturing a compassionate relationship with oneself, individuals can eat in accordance with their true desires and needs, promoting a more balanced and fulfilling relationship with food.

HOW TO DEAL WITH EMOTIONS WITHOUT EATING

Having a better awareness of emotional triggers and learning other coping strategies are essential to managing emotions without resorting to food for solace.

The first stage is awareness. Acknowledge the feelings causing the want for food. Determining the root cause of any emotional feeling, be it tension, boredom, melancholy, or worry, is essential to properly resolving it. Journaling and other mindfulness exercises can help people become more self-aware and be able to recognize their feelings without acting on them.

Examine more healthy coping mechanisms that provide solace and relief. Take part in joyful pursuits, such as hobbies, physical activity, or time spent in nature. For instance, engaging in physical exercise can release endorphins, which improve mood and reduce stress. Other effective ways to handle stress include muscle relaxation, deep breathing exercises, and seeking help through counseling or therapy. Create a support network. Reach out to friends, family, or support groups during times of emotional distress. Talking to someone supportive can provide comfort and perspective, offering an alternative outlet for processing emotions.

Make self-care routines part of an organized schedule. Make rest and relaxation a priority. Eat at regular intervals. Participate in things that help you feel good about yourself. Nurturing emotional wellness requires both establishing boundaries and engaging in self-compassion exercises.

It takes patience and work to build resilience so that you can control your emotions without eating. Throughout this path, it is essential to exercise patience and forgiveness toward oneself. A more balanced connection with food and emotions may be fostered by learning to sit with discomfort, acknowledge emotions without passing judgment, and develop healthy methods to confront and process feelings. These skills are essential to ending the cycle of emotional eating.

A healthy method to manage emotions is to express oneself creatively. Through self-expression via writing, music, art, or other creative endeavors, people can process and externalize their emotions in a healthy way.

And ultimately, it's critical to get expert assistance as needed. Counselors, therapists, and support groups provide direction and specialized techniques to deal with certain emotional problems. These materials offer helpful guidance and methods for effectively navigating and regulating emotions without resorting to food for solace. Without using food as a coping technique, people may build resilience and promote emotional well-being by combining self-awareness, healthy coping strategies, and seeking help.

Losing weight isn't about quick fixes, crash diets, or overnight transformations—it's about building habits that last a lifetime. Real, lasting change happens when you shift your mindset from "How fast can I lose weight?" to "How can I create a healthier lifestyle that I can stick with?"

Think of weight loss like a marathon, not a sprint. Some days will feel easy, like you're gliding forward effortlessly. Other days, you might feel stuck, frustrated, or even tempted to quit. And that's okay! The key isn't perfection—it's consistency.

Small, sustainable steps taken day after day will always win over extreme measures that burn you out.

The beauty of a long-term approach is that it allows you to enjoy the journey. You don't have to give up your favorite foods, punish yourself with endless workouts, or obsess over the scale. Instead, you'll learn how to balance nutrition, movement, and mindset in a way that feels natural and sustainable for YOU.

So, take a deep breath and remind yourself: You're not racing against the clock. You're building a healthier, happier future—one step, one meal, and one choice at a time.

Making long-term lifestyle adjustments that goes beyond diets is necessary to maintain weight loss. It's about developing long-term behaviors that promote a healthy weight and general wellbeing.

Prioritize first a healthy, well-balanced diet that fits your requirements and tastes. While limiting amounts, concentrate on complete, unprocessed meals that are high in fiber and nutrients. To avoid overindulging, practice mindful eating, paying attention to your hunger indicators, and enjoying your meals.

It's important to exercise regularly. Include fun exercises in your program; try to balance strength training, cardiovascular exercises, and mobility and flexibility-enhancing activities. Engage in activities or groups that promote a healthy lifestyle fosters motivation and accountability.

Building a network of support is really beneficial. Be in the company of people who support and encourage you in achieving your health objectives. Participating in events or gatherings

Maintaining consistency is essential. Create enduring habits for your sleep, diet, exercise, and stress reduction. Make sure your new habits are long-term sustainable by making sure they fit your lifestyle. Remind yourself not to give in to emotional eating cues. Create substitute coping mechanisms to handle boredom, stress, or emotions without eating. When faced with obstacles, practice self-compassion and resilience.

Review your objectives and track your progress on a regular basis. Celebrate successes and, if necessary, modify your strategy. Maintain a record of your routine, diet, and exercise to hold yourself responsible and make the required adjustments.

Consult a professional as required. Seek guidance from medical professionals, dietitians, or fitness specialists for individualized recommendations and needs based.

What's the biggest challenge you've faced in your weight loss journey so far, and how do you think a mindset shift could help?

If you could change just ONE small habit today to move toward a healthier lifestyle, what would it be? Why?

Think about a time when you tried to lose weight in the past—what worked well, and what didn't? How can you use those lessons moving forward?

In the book, we talked about sustainable weight loss being a long-term game. What's one long-term goal you'd love to achieve, and what's a small step you can take today to get there?

What's your relationship with food like?
Do you see it as fuel, comfort, or
something else? How can you create a
healthier, more balanced perspective?

Have you ever set weight loss goals that
felt overwhelming? How could you break
them down into smaller, more manageable
milestones?

What are three non-scale victories that would make you feel amazing on this journey? (Examples: having more energy, feeling stronger, fitting into old clothes, better sleep, etc.)

We often focus on what we "can't" eat when dieting. Instead, let's flip the script— what are some healthy foods you genuinely enjoy and can eat more of?

What is one way you can make movement and exercise feel fun rather than a chore? (Dancing? Hiking? Playing with your kids? Trying a new sport?)

If future-you could give you one piece of advice about staying consistent, what do you think they would say? How can you start applying that advice today?

The process of losing weight is just as important as the final result when trying to maintain it over time. Living a balanced, nourished, and thoughtful lifestyle creates the foundation for long-term success. It's about choosing decisions that put long-term health ahead of temporary cures, and cultivating a deep connection between body and mind. Recall that obstacles are a necessary part of the process as you proceed on this adventure. What counts most is your will to overcome setbacks with fortitude and a steadfast commitment to your health. You create the foundation for a rewarding, lifetime connection with health and vitality by incorporating healthy behaviors, creating a nurturing atmosphere, and adopting a holistic approach that supports both physical and emotional well. Appreciate the lessons you've learned, celebrate each accomplishment, and keep changing to become a more balanced, healthier version of yourself. It's important to adopt a lifestyle that feeds your body, mind, and spirit to ensure long-term health and satisfaction. Losing weight is only one aspect of this.